ANTI INFLAMMATORY RECIPES

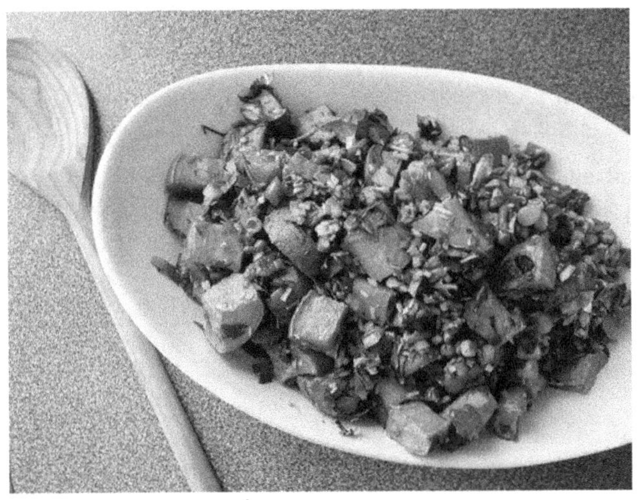

By Julia Bond

Copyright © 2017 by Julia Bond

The trademarks that are used are without any consent, and the publication of the trademark is without permission or backing by the trademark owner. All trademarks and brands within this book are for clarifying purposes only and are the owned by the owners themselves, not affiliated with this document.

Disclaimer and Terms of Use: The Author and Publisher has strived to be as accurate and complete as possible in the creation of this book, notwithstanding the fact that he does not warrant or represent at any time that the contents within are accurate due to the rapidly changing nature of the Internet. While all attempts have been made to verify information provided in this publication, the Author and Publisher assumes no responsibility for errors, omissions, or contrary interpretation of the subject matter herein.

Any perceived slights of specific persons, peoples, or organizations are unintentional. In practical advice books, like anything else in life, there are no guarantees of results. Readers are cautioned to rely on their own judgment about their individual circumstances and act accordingly.

This book is not intended for use as a source of legal, medical, business, accounting or financial advice. All readers are advised to seek services of competent professionals in the legal, medical, business, accounting, and finance fields.

TABLE OF CONTENTS

INTRODUCTION

Inflammation is a natural process with the biological purpose to initiate healing by increasing circulation. It is a complex process involving both the immune system and vascular system and the interplay of various chemical mediators. Increased circulation brings white blood cells and nourishment to the site of injury or infection so that invading pathogens are killed and damage may be repaired. Characteristic signs of inflammation include pain (dolor), heat (calor), swelling (tumor) and redness (rubor).

While some inflammation is beneficial and appropriate for healing, chronic or excessive inflammation, serving no purpose produces damage. Chronic inflammation has a bad reputation because it is implicated in various disease processes including (but not limited to)...

- autoimmune diseases

- arthritis

- diabetes

- Alzheimer's disease

- atherosclerosis (hardening of arteries that leads to heart attack and stroke)

- ADD and ADHD

- allergies & asthma

- cancers

- inflammatory bowel disease

Soft tissue swelling and chemical mediators involved in inflammation can also irritate nerve endings, contributing to pain.

It is a well-known fact that different foods are metabolized differently, some promoting inflammation and others reducing it.

The purpose of the anti-inflammatory diet is to promote optimal health and healing by choosing foods that reduce inflammation. If one can successfully control excessive inflammation through natural means (like through diet), it reduces one's dependence on anti-inflammatory medications that have unwanted and unhealthy side effects and don't solve the underlying problem. While anti-inflammatory medications (such as NSAIDs) are a quick fix to ease symptoms, they ultimately weaken the immune system by damaging the gastrointestinal tract which plays an important role in immune system function.

15 X BREAKFAST ANTI INFLAMMATORY RECIPES

Food plays an important role in controlling inflammation. We've put together a full week of recipes using foods that are known for their anti-inflammatory properties. Help manage your rheumatoid arthritis by eating right!

1. BREAKFAST: CHERRY COCONUT PORRIDGE

For a twist on traditional oatmeal porridge, add dried (or fresh) tart cherries. They contain anthocyanin, which is a powerful antioxidant that may help cut down inflammation.

CHERRY COCONUT PORRIDGE

- 1.5cups oats
- 4 tablespoons chia seed
- 3-4cups of coconut drinking milk
- 3 tablepoons raw cacao
- pinch of stevia
- coconut shavings
- cherries (fresh or frozen)
- dark chocolate shavings
- maple syrup

1. Combine oats, chia, coconut milk, cacao and stevia in a saucepan. Bring to a boil over medium heat and then simmer over lower heat until oats are cooked.

2. Pour into a bowl and top with coconut shavings, cherries, dark chocolate shavings and maple syrup to taste.

2. BREAKFAST: GINGERBREAD OATMEAL

Omega-3 fatty acids are a key ingredient in helping to reduce the inflammation of arthritis and other joint problems, but getting enough of it every day can be challenging. This oatmeal tastes great and gets you half your daily requirements of omega-3s — and no, we didn't add any salmon to it.

(Makes 4 servings)

INGREDIENTS:

- 4 cups water

- 1 cup steel cut oats

- 1 1/2 tablespoons ground cinnamon

- 1/4 teaspoon ground coriander

- 1 teaspoon ground cloves

- 1/4 teaspoon ground ginger

- 1/4 teaspoon ground allspice

- 1/8 teaspoon ground nutmeg

- 1/4 teaspoon ground cardamom

- Maple syrup to taste

DIRECTIONS:

1. Cook the oats to package directions but include the spices when you add the oats to the water.

2. When finished cooking, add maple syrup to taste.

3. BREAKFAST: RHUBARB, APPLE, AND GINGER MUFFINS

Not only does ginger taste great in these quick and easy gluten-free and dairy-free muffins, but it's also an excellent anti- inflammatory, helping to ease arthritis pain.

- 1/2 cup (55g) almond meal (ground almonds)

- 1/4 cup (50g) unrefined raw sugar

- 2 tablespoons finely chopped crystallised ginger

- 1 tablespoon ground linseed meal* see headnotes

- 1/2 cup (70g) buckwheat flour

- 1/4 cup (35g) fine brown rice flour

- 2 tablespoons organic cornflour or true arrowroot

- 2 teaspoons gluten-free baking powder

- 1/2 teaspoon ground cinnamon

- 1/2 teaspoon ground ginger

- a good pinch fine sea salt

- 1 cup finely sliced rhubarb

- 1 small apple, peeled, cored and finely diced

- 95ml (1/3 cup + 1 tablespoon) rice or almond milk

- 1/4 cup (60ml) olive oil

- 1 large free-range egg

- 1 teaspoon vanilla extract

INSTRUCTIONS

1. Preheat oven to 180C/350C. Grease or line eight 1/3 cup (80ml) cup capacity muffin tins with paper cases.

2. Place almond meal, sugar, ginger and linseed meal into a medium bowl. Sieve over flours, baking powder and spices, then whisk to combine evenly. Stir in rhubarb and apple to coat in the flour mixture. In another smaller bowl whisk milk, oil, egg and vanilla before pouring into the dry mixture and stirring until just combined. Evenly divide batter between tins/paper cases (scatter with a few slices of rhubarb if desired) and bake for 20-25 minutes or until risen, golden around the edges and when a skewer is inserted into the centre it comes out clean. Remove from the oven and set aside for 5 minutes before transferring to a wire rack to cool further. Eat warm or at room temperature Best eaten on the day of baking, however they will store in an airtight container for 2-3 days or frozen in zip-lock bags for longer.

4. BREAKFAST: BUCKWHEAT AND GINGER GRANOLA

Try this granola topped with almond milk or soy yogurt for an energizing breakfast.

I love this served with creamy coconut yoghurt and fresh berries, but it also tastes amazing mixed into a smoothie bowl or sprinkled over stewed fruit!

Makes one big container

- 2 cups of oats (220g)

- 1 cup of buckwheat (280g)

- 1 cup of sunflower seeds (200g)

- 1 cup of pumpkin seeds (200g)

- 1 and a ½ cups of pitted dates (300g)

- 1 cup of apple puree/sauce (about the size of a 360g jar)

- 6 tablespoons of coconut oil

- 4 tablesppons of raw cacao powder

- a piece of ginger (20g)

1. Start by pre-heating the oven to 180C

2. Then place the oats, buckwheat and seeds into a large mixing bowl and stir well

3. Next add the dates, coconut oil and apple puree into a sauce pan and allow them to simmer for five minutes, until the dates are nice and soft

4. While the dates cook peel the ginger and grate it onto a plate, once it's grated mix it into the date pan.

5. When the dates are soft place them (including the melted coconut oil, grated ginger and apple puree) into a blender with the raw cacao powder

and blend until the mix is totally smooth. Then pour the mix over the buckwheat, oat and seed mix and stir well so that everything is coated.

6. Grease one large or two medium baking trays with coconut oil before spreading the granola out over them

7. Place the baking trays in the oven and bake for about forty five minutes. After fifteen minutes remove the trays from the oven and stir everything well so that the top doesn't burn, then keep doing this every five to ten minutes for the rest of the time it's in the oven.

8. Once it's nice and crispy, but not burnt, take the granola out of the oven and allow it to cool before placing it in an airtight container to store. In an airtight container it will stay delicious for about a month or so.

5. BREAKFAST: GLUTEN-FREE CREPES

Many people think crepes are difficult to make. On the contrary, they're easy to prepare and a great way to make any meal special. Try filling these crepes with sliced strawberries or bananas. Alternately, you can make them for dinner and fill them with a stew or leftover chicken.

INGREDIENTS

- 2 eggs

- 1 teaspoon vanilla, gluten-free

- 1/2 cup nut milk

- 1/2 cup water

- 1/4 teaspoon salt

- 1-2 tablespoons agave nectar

- 1 cup gluten-free all purpose flour

- 2 tablespoons coconut oil, melted

- 1 tablespoon coconut oil, for pan

INSTRUCTIONS

1. Place 2 tablespoons of coconut oil into a small saucepan, and melt over low heat.

2. In a medium mixing bowl, whisk together the eggs, vanilla, nut milk, water, salt and agave nectar until combined.

3. Slowly add in the flour and whisk to combine.

4. Remove oil from heat, and pour into batter in a steady stream while slowly whisking to combine.

5. Mix until smooth.

6. Heat a small amount of coconut oil in a large frying pan over medium high heat.

7. Pour or scoop the batter onto the griddle, using approximately 1/3 cup for each crepe.

8. As soon as you've poured the batter, tilt and swirl the pan in a circular motion so that the batter coats the surface evenly.

9. Cook the crepe for about 2 minutes, until the bottom is light brown.

10. Flip the crepe with a spatula and cook the other side.

11. Repeat this process with remaining batter.

6. BREAK FAST: HOT OR CHILLED GINGER AND TURMERIC SPICED SPRING CARROT SOUP RECIPE

This bright, vibrantly spiced soup is velvety smooth and light. It's the essence of spring kicked up with a hit of heat, a little sunshine in a bowl.

Prep Time: 20 min

Cook Time: 25 min

INGREDIENTS

- 2 Tablespoons coconut oil

- 2 to 3 small green onions, white and light green parts only, cleaned and chopped

- 1 or 2 cloves of garlic, minced

- 1-inch piece of ginger, peeled and grated

- A pinch of red pepper flakes

- 1 ½ pounds young carrots, sliced 1/2 inch thick

- 1 tsp fine sea salt

- ¼ tsp ground cinnamon

- 1-inch piece of turmeric root, peeled and grated (or use ½ tsp ground)

- Freshly ground pepper to taste

- 4 cups (1 quart) filtered water

- ¼ cup plain yogurt or full fat coconut milk for serving

- Chopped flat leaf parsley or carrot fronds for garnish

INSTRUCTIONS

1. Melt coconut oil in a medium saucepan over medium heat. Sweat the green onions, garlic, minced ginger, and pepper flakes for 1 to 2 minutes or just until glossy. Do not brown or develop color.

2. Add carrots, salt, cinnamon and turmeric and cook another 1-2 minutes, stirring occasionally. Add water and bring to a boil. Reduce heat, and simmer until carrots are very soft, 20-25 minutes.

3. Puree soup in batches in a high speed blender.

4. If serving cold, chill soup for at least 3-4 hours or overnight.

5. Divide soup between 4 to 6 bowls and place a spoonful of yogurt or drizzle of coconut milk in center of each and finish with chopped parsley or carrot fonds and a pinch of additional salt and freshly ground pepper if desired.

7. BREAKFAST: GLOWING SPICED LENTIL SOUP

This soup is so quick and easy because there aren't many vegetables to chop (just garlic and onion—that's it!) and it relies mostly on pantry staples. It takes 15 minutes prep time (that includes getting the ingredients out), and then it's hands off while it cooks. Talk about easy! While this soup contains a lot of spices, it's not what I would call "spicy" or "hot". If you do want a kick of heat feel free to add some cayenne pepper or red pepper flakes. Also, feel free to change up the baby spinach for other greens like stemmed kale or chard. This soup is inspired by Whole Foods.

Yield: about 7 cups (1.65 litres)

Prep Time: 15 Minutes

Cook time: 20 Minutes

INGREDIENTS:

- 1 1/2 tablespoons extra-virgin olive oil

- 2 cups (280 grams) diced onion (1 medium/large)

- 2 large garlic cloves, minced

- 2 teaspoons ground turmeric

- 1 1/2 teaspoons ground cumin

- 1/2 teaspoon cinnamon

- 1/4 teaspoon ground cardamom

- 1 (15-ounce/398 mL) can diced tomatoes, with juices

- 1 (15-ounce/398 mL) can full-fat coconut milk*

- 3/4 cup (140 grams) uncooked red lentils, rinsed and drained

- 3 1/2 cups (875 mL) low-sodium vegetable broth

- 1/2 teaspoon fine sea salt, or to taste

- Freshly ground black pepper, to taste

- Red pepper flakes or cayenne pepper, to taste (for a kick of heat!)

- 1 (5-ounce/140-gram) package baby spinach

- 2 teaspoons fresh lime juice, or more to taste

DIRECTIONS:

1. In a large pot, add the oil, onion, and garlic. Add a pinch of salt, stir, and sauté over medium heat for 4 to 5 minutes until the onion softens.

2. Stir in the turmeric, cumin, cinnamon, and cardamom until combined. Continue cooking for about 1 minute, until fragrant.

3. Add the diced tomatoes (with juices), entire can of coconut milk, red lentils, broth, salt, and plenty of pepper. Add red pepper flakes or cayenne, if desired, to taste. Stir to combine. Increase heat to high and bring to a low boil.

4. Once it boils, reduce the heat to medium-high, and simmer, uncovered, for about 18 to 22 minutes, until the lentils are fluffy and tender.

5. Turn off the heat and stir in the spinach until wilted. Add the lime juice to taste. Taste and add more salt and pepper, if desired. Ladle into bowls and serve with toasted bread and lime wedges.

8. VEGAN TURMERIC QUINOA POWER BOWLS

Cook Time: 30 minutes

Total Time: 30 minutes

Servings: 4

Calories: 385 kcal

INGREDIENTS

- 7 small yellow potatoes

- 15 oz . can chickpeas

- 2 tsp turmeric

- 1 tsp paprika

- 1 Tbsp coconut oil

- 1/4 cup quinoa

- salt/pepper

- 2 kale leaves

- 1/2 Tbsp olive oil

- 1 avocado

INSTRUCTIONS

1. Preheat oven to 350 degrees.

2. Slice the potatoes into strips and lay flat on 1/2 of a baking sheet. Spray/ drizzle them with coconut oil and sprinkle 1 tsp of turmeric over them. Add salt/pepper to taste.

3. Roast for 5 minutes while you drain and rinse the chickpeas.

4. Place the chickpeas in a mixing bowl and add 1 tsp of paprika, coating them evenly. Lay the chickpeas on the other 1/2 of the baking sheet.

5. Roast the chickpeas and the potatoes for about 25 minutes (or until the potatoes are a little bit soft).

6. Cook the quinoa with 1/2 cup of water. Once the quinoa is cooked, add 1 tsp of turmeric (salt/pepper to taste), mix together, and let cool.

7. Wash the kale and massage the olive oil over the leaves. Separate the leaves into the 4 bowls.

8. Slice the avocado and split into the 4 bowls.

9. Add the quinoa and roasted chickpeas/potatoes to the bowls and serve!

9. TURMERIC OATMEAL - A GLOWING BREAKFAST BOWL

Turmeric Oatmeal gives your breakfast a super health kick. With its anti-inflammatory properties, turmeric is a great addition to your diet. Try it out in this unique, delicious breakfast recipe!

Course: Breakfast

Cuisine: Vegan

Prep Time: 5 minutes

Cook Time: 15 minutes

Servings: 1

INGREDIENTS

- Oatmeal

- 1/2 cup Whole Rolled Oats

- 1 cup Water

- 1 splash Oat Milk or any other plant milk you like

- 1/2 teaspoon Turmeric Powder

Toppings

- Raspberries
- Bluberries
- Mixed Seeds
- Flaked Almonds
- Dried Cranberries
- Desiccated Coconut
- Mint Leaves
- Maple Syrup optional

10. BLUEBERRY YOGURT SMOOTHIE

Prep Time: 5 Minutes

Difficulty: Easy

Servings: 1 Servings

INGREDIENTS

- 1 cup Plain, Unflavored Yogurt

- 1 cup Fruit (your Choice - Blueberries, Peaches, Pineapple, Etc)

- 1/4 cup Milk

- 1 dash Honey

- Ice

INSTRUCTIONS

1. Place yogurt, fruit, milk, a handful of ice and honey to taste all into a blender. Blend until smooth. Taste it for sweetness and add more honey if needed.

2. Pour, drink and enjoy!

11. GOLDEN MILK ICE CREAM

Prep time: 8 hours

Cook time: 5 mins

Total time: 8 hours 5 mins

A creamy, coconut milk-based ice cream inspired by Golden Milk! Ground turmeric, cinnamon, black pepper, ginger, and cardamom bring plenty of rich, warm flavor to this insanely delicious ice cream.

Recipe type: Dessert

Cuisine: Vegan, Gluten-Free

Serves: 8

INGREDIENTS

- 2 14-ounce (414 ml) cans full-fat coconut milk, (~3 1/2 cups or 840 ml | sub coconut cream for even creamier ice cream!)

- 4 quarter-size slices fresh ginger

- 1/4 cup (60 ml) maple syrup (sub up to half with organic cane sugar), plus more to taste

- Pinch sea salt

- 2 tsp ground turmeric

- 1/2 tsp ground cinnamon

- 1/8th tsp black pepper

- optional: 1/8th tsp cardamom

- 1 tsp pure vanilla extract

- optional: 2 Tbsp (30 ml) olive oil

- optional: 1/4 cup chopped candied ginger

INSTRUCTIONS

1. The day or night before, place your ice cream churning bowl in the freezer to properly chill (see notes if you don't have an ice cream maker). Also, add coconut milk, fresh ginger, maple syrup, sea salt, turmeric, cinnamon, pepper, and cardamom (optional) to a large saucepan and heat over medium heat.

2. Bring to a simmer (not a boil), whisking to thoroughly combine ingredients. Then, remove from heat and add vanilla extract. Whisk once more to combine.

3. Taste and adjust flavor as needed, adding in more turmeric for intense turmeric flavor, cinnamon for warmth, maple syrup for sweetness, or salt to balance the flavors.

4. Transfer mixture (including the whole ginger slices) to a mixing bowl and let cool to room temperature. Then cover and chill in refrigerator overnight, or for at least 4-6 hours.

5. The following day, use a spoon (or strainer) to remove the ginger. At this time, you can also add olive oil for extra creaminess by whisking in thoroughly to combine (optional).

6. Add to ice cream maker and churn according to manufacturer's instructions - about 20-30 minutes. It should look like soft serve.

7. While it's churning, chop up your candied ginger (optional). In the last few minutes of churning, add in the ginger to incorporate.

8. Once churned, transfer the ice cream to a large freezer-safe container (such as a parchment-lined loaf pan) and use a spoon to smooth the top.

9. Cover securely and freeze for at least 4-6 hours or until firm. Set out for 10 minutes before serving to soften, and use a hot ice cream scoop (warmed in hot water) to ease scooping.

10. Will keep in the freezer for up to 10 days or more, though best within the first 7 days. Enjoy this as a lighter dessert with some serious health benefits!

12. ANTI-INFLAMMATORY HOT CHOCOLATE

Difficulty: easy

Cooking time: less than 15 minutes

Serves: 1

INGREDIENTS

- 1 tablespoon raw cacao powder
- ½ teaspoon cinnamon
- ¼ teaspoon dried ginger
- ½ teaspoon dried turmeric (depending on your taste)
- pinch of cayenne pepper
- pinch of cardamom (optional)
- teaspoon rice malt syrup, to taste (we recommend no more than 1/2 teaspoon)
- pinch of sea salt and freshly ground black pepper
- ½ cup coconut milk, warmed
- ½ cup water

INSTRUCTION

1. Add raw cacao powder, dried spices, sea salt and pepper into a standard mug.

2. Fill mug halfway with boiling water and rice malt syrup and stir until powders dissolve.

3. Pour in warmed coconut milk and stir to combine.

4. Serve warm.

13. RED LENTIL SOUP WITH LEMON

This is a lentil soup that defies expectations of what lentil soup can be. It is light, spicy and a bold red color (no murky brown here): a revelatory dish that takes less than an hour to make. The cooking is painless. Sauté onion and garlic in oil, then stir in tomato paste, cumin and chile powder and cook a few minutes more to intensify flavor. Add broth, water, red lentils (which cook faster than their green or black counterparts) and diced carrot, and simmer for 30 minutes. Purée half the mixture and return it to the pot for a soup that strikes the balance between chunky and pleasingly smooth. A hit of lemon juice adds an up note that offsets the deep cumin and chile flavors.

INGREDIENTS

- 3 tablespoons olive oil, more for drizzling

- 1 large onion, chopped

- 2 garlic cloves, minced

- 1 tablespoon tomato paste

- 1 teaspoon ground cumin

- ¼ teaspoon kosher salt, more to taste

- ¼ teaspoon ground black pepper

- Pinch of ground chile powder or cayenne, more to taste

- 1 quart chicken or vegetable broth

- 2 cups water

- 1 cup red lentils

- 1 large carrot, peeled and diced

- Juice of 1/2 lemon, more to taste

- 3 tablespoons chopped fresh cilantro

PREPARATION

Step 1

In a large pot, heat 3 tablespoons oil over high heat until hot and shimmering. Add onion and garlic, and sauté until golden, about 4 minutes.

Step 2

Stir in tomato paste, cumin, salt, black pepper and chili powder or cayenne, and sauté for 2 minutes longer.

Step 3

Add broth, 2 cups water, lentils and carrot. Bring to a simmer, then partially cover pot and turn heat to medium-low. Simmer until lentils are soft, about 30 minutes. Taste and add salt if necessary.

Step 4

Using an immersion or regular blender or a food processor, purée half the soup then add it back to pot. Soup should be somewhat chunky.

Step 5

Reheat soup if necessary, then stir in lemon juice and cilantro. Serve soup drizzled with good olive oil and dusted lightly with chili powder if desired.

14. THE LIFE-CHANGING LOAF OF BREAD

Makes 1 loaf

INGREDIENTS:

- 1 cup / 135g sunflower seeds

- ½ cup / 90g flax seeds

- ½ cup / 65g hazelnuts or almonds

- 1 ½ cups / 145g rolled oats

- 2 Tbsp. chia seeds

- 4 Tbsp. psyllium seed husks (3 Tbsp. if using psyllium husk powder)

- 1 tsp. fine grain sea salt (add ½ tsp. if using coarse salt)

- 1 Tbsp. maple syrup (for sugar-free diets, use a pinch of stevia)

- 3 Tbsp. melted coconut oil or ghee

- 1 ½ cups / 350ml water

DIRECTIONS:

1. In a flexible, silicon loaf pan combine all dry ingredients, stirring well. Whisk maple syrup, oil and water together in a measuring cup. Add this to the dry ingredients and mix very well until everything is completely soaked and dough becomes very thick (if the dough is too thick to stir, add one or two teaspoons of water until the dough is manageable). Smooth out the top with the back of a spoon. Let sit out on the counter for at least 2 hours, or all day or overnight. To ensure the dough is ready, it should retain its shape even when you pull the sides of the loaf pan away from it it.

2. Preheat oven to 350°F / 175°C.

3. Place loaf pan in the oven on the middle rack, and bake for 20 minutes.

Remove bread from loaf pan, place it upside down directly on the rack and bake for another 30-40 minutes. Bread is done when it sounds hollow when tapped. Let cool completely before slicing (difficult, but important).

4. Store bread in a tightly sealed container for up to five days. Freezes well too – slice before freezing for quick and easy toast!

15. CHILI PUMPKIN SOUP

Pumpkins are an excellent source of beta-cryptoxanthin, a powerful anti-inflammatory. This antioxidant is absorbed best when paired with a fat, making the butter and oil in this recipe important for more than just flavor. Pumpkin skins are edible which makes preparing this soup very easy! Serve this soup with a mixed green salad for a healthy lunch or as the first course of a holiday dinner.

INGREDIENTS

- 1 tablespoon olive oil

- 1 red onion, chopped

- 3 garlic cloves, crushed

- 2 (300g) golden delight potatoes, peeled, chopped

- 1kg butternut pumpkin, peeled, chopped

- 1/4 teaspoon dried chilli flakes

- 2 teaspoons ground coriander

- 1 litre salt-reduced chicken stock

- 1/2 cup pure cream

- Pure cream, to serve

- Chopped fresh chives, to serve

- Toast, to serve

METHOD

Step 1

Heat oil in a saucepan over medium-high heat. Add onion and garlic. Cook, stirring, for 3 minutes or until onion has softened. Add potato and pumpkin. Cook, stirring occasionally, for 5 minutes or until potato starts to brown. Add chilli and coriander. Cook for 1 minute or until fragrant.

Step 2

Add stock. Cover. Bring to the boil. Reduce heat to medium-low. Simmer for 10 to 12 minutes or until potato and pumpkin are tender. Set aside for 2 minutes to cool slightly.

Step 3

Blend in batches until smooth. Return to pan over low heat. Stir in cream. Cook for 1 minute or until heated through. Season with pepper. Divide between bowls. Top with cream and chives. Serve with toast.

15 LUNCH ANTI INFLAMMATORY RECIPES

1. MEDITERRANEAN TUNA SALAD

Tuna is an excellent source of omega-3 fatty acids. Serve it on top of mixed greens or spread onto whole grain bread. This recipe is high sodium, so you can scale it back by choosing low sodium canned tuna, and by reducing the amount of capers and olives.

INGREDIENTS

Serves: 2

- 2, 5oz cans tuna packed in water, drained

- 1/4 cup mayonnaise

- 1/4 cup chopped kalamata or mixed olives

- 2 Tablespoons minced red onion

- 2 Tablespoons chopped fire roasted red peppers

- 2 Tablespoons chopped fresh basil

- 1 Tablespoon capers

- 1 Tablespoon fresh lemon juice

- salt and pepper

- 2 large vine-ripened tomatoes

DIRECTIONS

Add all ingredients except tomatoes in a large bowl then stir to combine. Slice tomatoes into sixths, without cutting all the way through, then gently pry open. Scoop Mediterranean Tuna Salad mixture into the center then serve.

Notes: Could also serve tuna salad as a sandwich, in a pita pocket, on a bed of greens, or with crackers.

2. LUNCH: KALE CAESAR SALAD WITH GRILLED CHICKEN WRAP

Whole roasted chicken, often found in the neighborhood supermarket, is a great time saver for quick meals. Pick up two — one for dinner that evening and another for these tasty lunch wraps. They're perfect to toss into your lunch bag. If avoiding gluten, choose a gluten-free wrap.

INGREDIENTS

1. 8 ounces grilled chicken, thinly sliced

2. 6 cups curly kale, cut into bite sized pieces

3. 1 cup cherry tomatoes, quartered

4. 3/4 cup finely shredded Parmesan cheese

5. ½ coddled egg (cooked about 1 minute)

6. 1 clove garlic, minced

7. 1/2 teaspoon Dijon mustard

8. 1 teaspoon honey or agave

9. 1/8 cup fresh lemon juice

10. 1/8 cup olive oil

11. Kosher salt and freshly ground black pepper

12. 2 Lavash flat breads or two large tortillas

INSTRUCTIONS

1. In a bowl, mix together the half of a coddled egg, minced garlic, mustard, honey, lemon juice and olive oil. Whisk until you have formed a dressing. Season to taste with salt and pepper.

2. Add the kale, chicken and cherry tomatoes and toss to coat with the dressing and ¼ cup of the shredded parmesan.

3. Spread out the two lavash flatbreads. Evenly distribute the salad over the two wraps and sprinkle each with ¼ cup of parmesan.

4. Roll up the wraps and slice in half. Eat immediately

Preparation time: 10 minute(s)

Number of servings (yield): 2

3. WINTER FRUIT SALAD

If you're taking this salad to work, you'll want to keep the fruit separate from the dressing. Otherwise, it will saturate and soften the fruit too much. Toss the remaining ingredients into a separate container. When you're ready to eat, simply mix it all together!

Winter Fruit Salad with Persimmons, Pears, Grapes, Pecans, and Agave-Pomegranate Vinaigrette (Makes about 6 side-dish servings, recipe created by Kalyn with inspiration from Local Flavors by Deborah Madison.)

INGREDIENTS:

- 4 Fuyu persimmons, cut in 1 inch cubes (or enough cut persimmons to make 2 cups)

- 3 Bosch pears, cut in 1 inch cubes (or enough cut pears to make 2 cups)

- 1 cup grapes, cut into halves or fourths if large (I would have used more grapes if I'd had more)

- (Other fruits such as apples, figs, or pomegranate arils could be used to replace any of these, but you need 5-6 cups of cut fruit)

- 3/4 cup pecans, cut into half lengthwise to make slivers

DRESSING INGREDIENTS:

- 1 T extra virgin olive oil (use a fruity oil for this)

- 1 T peanut oil

- 1 T pomegranate-flavored vinegar (I used pomegranate-flavored red wine vinegar)

- 2 T agave nectar
  (If you have pomegranate molasses I might use white balsamic vinegar and substitute pomegranate molasses for some or all of the agave nectar)

- pinch of salt, to taste

INSTRUCTIONS:

Whisk together the dressing ingredients so flavors can blend while you cut the fruit.

Cut grapes, persimmons, and pears into same size pieces (about 1 inch size) and place in plastic bowl. Toss fruit with dressing. Just before serving, toss with pecan pieces.

4. ROASTED RED PEPPER AND SWEET POTATO SOUP

This antioxidant-rich soup freezes easily so you can prepare it ahead for the week. Roasting the sweet potatoes before simmering will make the flavors more pronounced. To reduce the sodium, try fresh roasted red peppers instead of the jarred version.

Prep time: 25 mins

Cook time: 30 mins

Total time: 55 mins

INGREDIENTS

- 2 tablespoons olive oil

- 2 medium onions, chopped

- 1 jar (12 oz) roasted red peppers, chopped, liquid reserved

- 1 can (4 oz) diced green chiles

- 2 teaspoons ground cumin

- 1 teaspoon salt

- 1 teaspoon ground coriander

- 3 - 4 cups peeled, cubed sweet potatoes

- 4 cups vegetable broth

- 2 tablespoons minced fresh cilantro

- 1 tablespoon lemon juice

- 4 oz cream cheese, cubed

INSTRUCTIONS

1. In a large soup pot or Dutch oven, heat the olive oil over medium-high heat. Add the onion and cook until soft. Add in the red peppers, green chiles, cumin, salt and coriander. Cook for 1-2 minutes.

2. Stir in the reserved juice from the roasted red peppers, sweet potatoes and vegetable broth. Bring to a boil, then reduce heat and cover. Cook until the potatoes are tender, 10-15 minutes. Stir in the cilantro and lemon juice. Let the soup cool slightly.

3. Place half of the soup into a blender along with the cream cheese. Process until smooth, then add back into the soup pot and heat through. Season with additional salt, if needed.

5. ROASTED RED PEPPER AND SWEET POTATO SOUP

This antioxidant-rich soup freezes easily so you can prepare it ahead for the week. Roasting the sweet potatoes before simmering will make the flavors more pronounced. To reduce the sodium, try fresh roasted red peppers instead of the jarred version.

Prep time: 25 mins

Cook time: 30 mins

Total time: 55 mins

Roasted red peppers and sweet potatoes come together in this creamy soup that is full of flavor.

Serves: 6 servings

INGREDIENTS

- 2 tablespoons olive oil

- 2 medium onions, chopped

- 1 jar (12 oz) roasted red peppers, chopped, liquid reserved

- 1 can (4 oz) diced green chiles

- 2 teaspoons ground cumin

- 1 teaspoon salt

- 1 teaspoon ground coriander

- 3 - 4 cups peeled, cubed sweet potatoes

- 4 cups vegetable broth

- 2 tablespoons minced fresh cilantro

- 1 tablespoon lemon juice

- 4 oz cream cheese, cubed

INSTRUCTIONS

1. In a large soup pot or Dutch oven, heat the olive oil over medium-high heat. Add the onion and cook until soft. Add in the red peppers, green chiles, cumin, salt and coriander. Cook for 1-2 minutes.

2. Stir in the reserved juice from the roasted red peppers, sweet potatoes and vegetable broth. Bring to a boil, then reduce heat and cover. Cook until the potatoes are tender, 10-15 minutes. Stir in the cilantro and lemon juice. Let the soup cool slightly.

3. Place half of the soup into a blender along with the cream cheese. Process until smooth, then add back into the soup pot and heat through. Season with additional salt, if needed.

6. SMOKED SALMON POTATO TARTINE

More omega-3s, please. Trade in the tuna for salmon and serve with a green salad or a cup of soup for a filling meal.

INGREDIENTS:

Potato Tartine:

- 1 large russet potato, peeled and grated lengthwise

- 2 tablespoons clarified butter (or other neutral flavored oil)

- salt

- pepper

Toppings:

- 4 ounces soft goat cheese, at room temperature

- 1 1/2 tablespoons finely minced chives

- 1/2 garlic clove, finely minced

- zest of half a lemon

- thinly sliced smoked salmon

- 2 tablespoons drained capers

- 2 tablespoons finely chopped red onion

- 1/2 hard boiled egg, finely chopped

- finely minced chives (for garnish)

DIRECTIONS:

Assemble Toppings:

1. Combine goat cheese, lemon zest, and garlic in small bowl. Season with salt and pepper to taste. Gently stir in fresh chives. Set aside.

2. Season the chopped red onion and hard-boiled egg with salt.

Prepare Potato Tartine:

1. Working quickly (as the potato will quickly begin to oxidize), grate the potato (lengthwise) into a large using the large holes of a grater. Squeeze the potatoes over the sink to remove any excess liquid. Season generously with salt and pepper and toss.

2. Heat clarified butter in a 8-10 inch non-stick skillet over medium-high heat. Once hot, add the grated potato and shape roughly, using a spatula, into a large circle.

3. Press on the mixture with the back of a spoon to compact it, cover and cook gently for 8-10 minutes or until the bottom is golden brown.

4. Flip carefully to other side and cook for another 8-10 minutes or until golden brown and crispy. Remove to cooling rack and allow to cool until barely lukewarm or room temperature.

Assemble Tartine:

1. Once potato cake has cooled, spread the goat cheese mixture on the top. Layer the smoked salmon directly over this and sprinkle with the red onion, hard-boiled egg, and capers. Garnish with freshly chopped chives.

2. Cut into wedges and serve immediately.

7. RED LENTIL AND SQUASH CURRIED STEW

This is a great make-ahead soup. Simply portion into single servings, freeze, and then pop one into your lunch sack for work. It should be thawed out enough to reheat in the microwave when lunchtime rolls around.

Yield: ~4 servings

INGREDIENTS:

- 1 tsp Extra virgin olive oil

- 1 sweet onion, chopped

- 3 garlic cloves, minced

- 1 tbsp good quality curry powder (or more to taste)

- 1 carton broth (4 cups) I used low-sodium

- 1 cup red lentils

- 3 cups cooked butternut squash

- 1 cup greens of choice

- Fresh grated ginger, to taste (optional)

- Kosher salt & black pepper, to taste (I used about 1/2 tsp salt)

1. In a large pot, add EVOO and chopped onion and minced garlic. Sautee for about 5 minutes over low-medium heat.

2. Stir in curry powder and cook another couple minutes. Add broth and lentils and bring to a boil. Reduce heat and cook for 10 minutes.

3. Stir in cooked butternut squash and greens of choice. Cook over medium heat for about 5-8 minutes. Season with salt, pepper, and add some freshly grated ginger to taste.

8. ANTI-INFLAMMATORY MEATBALLS

INGREDIENTS:

- 5 pounds grass-fed ground beef

- 5 garlic cloves, chopped

- 1/2 tsp turmeric

- 1/2 tsp ginger

- 1/4 tsp sea salt

DIRECTIONS:

1. Mix ground meat in a medium-sized bowl with chopped garlic, ginger, turmeric, and sea salt.

2. Once everything is sufficiently mixed, section the meat into 1 1/2 inch balls and place in an oven-safe dish.

3. Bake at 350F for 30-35 minutes until cooked all the way through.

4. For AIP or Low-Carb pair it with sauteed spinach or spaghetti squash.

9. COCONUT, CHAI & TURMERIC CHIA PUDDING

INGREDIENTS

- 5 tablespoons chia seeds.

- 1 tablespoon shredded coconut.

- 1 1/2 cup Pureharvest Organic Oat Milk.

- 1/4 teaspoon pure vanilla essence or powder.

- 1 teaspoon ground turmeric.

- 1/8 teaspoon ground cloves.

- 1/8 teaspoon ground cardamom.

- 1/2 teaspoon ground cinnamon.

Optional

- 1 tablespoon Pureharvest Organic Rice Malt Syrup.

DIRECTIONS

1. Mix the dry ingredients in a bowl, making sure no clumps of spices remain.

2. Add oat milk, vanilla essence and rice malt syrup, stirring until combined.

3. Cover and leave in fridge overnight to set.

4. Serve as is or top with chopped nuts and more shredded coconut.

10. ONE-SHEET ROASTED GARLIC SALMON & BROCCOLI

Serves: 4

INGREDIENTS:

1. 1 1/2 pounds salmon fillets, skinned and cut into 4 portions

2. 2 heads of broccoli, washed and cut into florets (about 4 cups)

3. 3 tablespoons avocado oil or melted coconut oil

4. 1-2 cloves of garlic, minced and divided

5. 1 1/4 teaspoon of sea salt, divided

6. 1/2 teaspoon ground black pepper, divided

7. 1 sliced lemon (optional)

DIRECTIONS:

1. Preheat oven to 450F and line a large baking sheet with parchment paper or a silicon baking mat.

2. Arrange the salmon pieces on the lined baking sheet, leaving a few inches between the portions. Drizzle 1 tablespoon of oil over the fish. Spread the minced garlic cloves evenly over the salmon next. Next, sprinkle the fish with 1/2 teaspoon salt and 1/4 teaspoon ground black pepper. Finally, arrange the sliced lemon (if using) on top of the salmon pieces.

3. Next, combine the clean broccoli florets 2 tablespoons of oil, 3/4 teaspoon sea salt and 1/4 teaspoon ground black pepper in a medium bowl. Toss to evenly coat the florets. Arrange the broccoli on the baking sheet around the salmon pieces.

4. Bake in the oven for 13-15 minutes or until fish is done and the broccoli florets are slightly golden on the ends.

5. Enjoy warm.

11. FRESH SPINACH MUSHROOM FRITTATA

Similar to omelettes or quiches, frittatas provide a backdrop for an endless combination of ingredients. In this case, we're using nutrient-rich mushrooms and spinach that are both bursting with flavor.

INGREDIENTS NUTRITION

Servings: 2-3

- 2 tablespoons butter
- 3 cloves garlic, minced
- 1/2 cup onion, sliced
- 8 ounces mushrooms, quartered
- 2 cups fresh spinach, chopped
- 6 eggs
- 1/2 teaspoon salt
- 1 dash pepper
- 1/2 cup grated parmesan cheese

DIRECTIONS

1. Melt butter in an oven proof skillet.
2. Add garlic, onions and mushrooms cooking until onions are translucent.
3. Add spinach, sautee for 2 minutes.
4. Beat eggs, salt& pepper together.
5. Pour over mixture in skillet, stirring to combine.
6. Cook eggs for about 4 minutes, eggs will be almost but not quite set still moist on top.
7. Sprinkle with cheese and put in oven.
8. Broil 6" from heat for 3-4 minutes or until eggs are set and cheese is lightly browned.

12. BEET AND CITRUS SALAD WITH PINE NUT VINAIGRETTE RECIPE

Yield: Serves 4 to 6

Active Time: 30 minutes

Total Time: 2 hours

INGREDIENTS

1. 2 pounds raw beets, greens and stems removed, scrubbed under cold running water

2. 5 tablespoons extra-virgin olive oil, divided

3. Kosher salt and freshly ground black pepper

4. 4 sprigs rosemary or thyme

5. 2 tablespoons sherry vinegar

6. 1 tablespoon agave nectar (or honey, for non-vegan version)

7. 1/4 cup toasted pinenuts, divided

8. 1 small shallot, finely minced, about 1 tablespoon

9. 1 tablespoon walnut oil

10. 1 grapefruit, cut into segments

11. 1 orange, cut into segments

12. 1 cup loosely packed arugula leaves

13. Orange zest, for garnish

DIRECTIONS

1. Adjust oven rack to middle position and preheat oven to 375°F. Fold two 12- by 18-inch squares of heavy duty aluminum foil in half cross-wise. Crimp the left and right edges to form a tight seal (leave the top open). Toss beets with 1 tablespoon olive oil and season with salt and pepper. Divide evenly between both foil pouches. Add 2 sprigs rosemary or thyme to each pouch, then tightly crimp top of pouch to seal.

2. Place pouches on a rimmed baking sheet and place in oven. Cook until beets are completely tender and a cake tester or toothpick inserted into a beet through the foil pouch shows no resistance, about 1 hour. Open pouches and allow beets to cool for 30 minutes. Peel under cold running water (the skin should slip right off). Cut beets into rough 1 1/2-inch chunks.

3. Combine vinegar, agave nectar, half of pinenuts, and shallots in a medium bowl. Whisking constantly, slowly drizzle in remaining 4 tablespoons olive oil followed by walnut oil. Season dressing to taste with salt and pepper.

4. Toss beets with half of dressing in a large bowl, then transfer to a serving plate. Add grapefruit, orange, and arugula leaves to bowl along with 1 more tablespoon dressing. Toss and season to taste with salt and pepper. Transfer to serving plate with beets. Drizzle remaining dressing around beets, sprinkle with remaining pinenuts, top with orange zest, and serve.

13. CREAMY BEET, CARROT & POTATO SOUP

INGREDIENTS

- 5 carrots

- 1 raw beetroot (not the cooked kind if you can help it)

- 2 sticks of celery

- 1 sweet potato

- 1 tbsp. of turmeric

- 1 thumb sized piece of ginger, grated or chopped finely.

- 1 garlic clove chopped.

- 1 tablespoon of vegan bouillon powder (or a powdered stock cube that has no MSG, Gluten or dairy)

- 1 tablespoon

- 1 tablespoon of coconut cream or a dairy free alternative

STEPS

1. Wash and chop all the vegetables and place in boiling water. Then add the ginger, garlic, turmeric and bouillon powder.

2. Once boiled, cover and simmer on a low heat and cook for 25 minutes.

3. Once vegetables are soft, allow to cool for ten minutes.

4. Add ingredients to your blender (I used my trusty nutribullet), alongside coconut cream/dairy free milk alternative to add creaminess (note coconut cream will make it extra creamy, milk alternatives will make it slightly thinner) and blend for 30 seconds.

5. For an extra health kick sprinkle with protein Powder (I used my That's Protein pumpkin/chia seed powder but you could also use flaxseed powder.)

6. Serve with seed crackers or a hearty dose of gluten free bread!

14. ROASTED GOLDEN BEETS WITH ROSEMARY AND GARLIC

Roasted Golden Beets with Rosemary and Garlic. The herbs and garlic enhance the sweetness and flavor of these delicious beets.

Prep Time: 10 minutes

Cook Time: 40 minutes

Total Time: 50 minutes

Servings: 4

INGREDIENTS

- 6 inch medium golden beets peeled and cut into 1- chunks (red beets are a perfectly good substitution)

- 3 cloves garlic minced or crushed

- 1 tbsp rosemary finely chopped (if using dry, use 1 tsp)

- Salt and black pepper to taste

- 2 tbsp extra virgin olive oil

INSTRUCTIONS

1. Preheat the oven to 400 degrees F

2. Mix together the garlic, rosemary, olive oil and salt and pepper.

3. In a bowl, place the beets and toss them with the herb-olive-oil mixture.

4. Spread in a single layer on a baking sheet, preferably coated with aluminum foil to make cleanup easier, and roast 35-40 minutes or until the beets are fork tender and golden. Stir once or twice during roasting to make sure they cook evenly.

5. Serve hot or cold.

15. RICH BEET & CHOCOLATE PUDDING

INGREDIENTS

- 2 large ripe avocados peeled and diced

- 1/2 cup raw cacao powder or unsweetened cocoa powder

- 1/2 cup red beet roasted

- 1/2 cup full-fat canned coconut milk

- 1/3 cup pure maple syrup

- 1/2 teaspoon ground cinnamon

- 1/8 teaspoon sea salt

INSTRUCTIONS

1. Add all of the ingredients for the pudding to a food processor. Process until completely smooth. Note: you may need to stop the food processor a couple times to scrape the sides and re-start to get it to a smooth consistency.

2. Transfer pudding to a sealable container and refrigerate until chilled. Serve with coconut whipped cream on top!

15 DINNER ANTI INFLAMMATORY RECIPES

1. CURRIED POTATOES WITH POACHED EGGS

Eggs aren't just for breakfast! Serve them poached with potatoes and a fresh garden salad for a nutritious dinner. If poached eggs aren't your thing, try sautéing them in a nonstick skillet. Eggs from pastured hens or those purchased from farmers markets are typically higher in omega-3 fatty acids, known anti-inflammatory fats.

It only takes a few ingredients to make these simple and flavorful Curried Potatoes with Poached Eggs. Perfect for brunch or dinner.

Prep Time: 10 minutes

Cook Time: 30 minutes

Total Time: 40 minutes

Servings: 4

INGREDIENTS

- 2 russet potatoes (about 2 lbs.) $2.09

- 1 inch fresh ginger $0.39

- 2 cloves garlic $0.16

- 1 Tbsp olive oil $0.16

- 2 Tbsp curry powder (hot or mild) $0.60

- 15 oz can tomato sauce $0.89

- 4 large eggs $0.76

- 1/2 bunch fresh cilantro (optional) $0.34

INSTRUCTIONS

1. Wash the potatoes well, then cut into 3/4-inch cubes. Place the cubed potatoes in a large pot and cover with water. Cover the pot with a lid and bring it up to a boil over high heat. Boil the potatoes for 5-6 minutes, or until they're tender when pierced with a fork. Drain the cooked potatoes in a colander.

2. While the potatoes are boiling, begin the sauce. Peel the ginger with a vegetable peeler or scrape the skin off with the side of a spoon. Use a small holed cheese grater to grate about one inch of ginger (less if you prefer a more subtle ginger flavor). Mince the garlic.

3. Add the ginger, garlic, and olive oil to a large, deep skillet (or a wide based pot). Sauté the ginger and garlic over medium low heat for 1-2 minutes, or just until soft and fragrant. Add the curry powder to the skillet and sauté for about a minute more to toast the spices.

4. 4. Add the tomato sauce to the skillet and stir to combine. Turn the heat up to medium and heat the sauce through. Taste the sauce and add salt, if needed. Add the cooked and drained potatoes to the skillet and stir to coat in the sauce. Add a couple tablespoons of water if the mixture seems dry or pasty.

5. Create four small wells or dips in the potato mixture and crack an egg into each. Place a lid on the skillet and let it come up to a simmer. Simmer the eggs in the sauce for 6-10 minutes, or until cooked through (less time if runny yolks are desired). Top with chopped fresh cilantro.

If you don't have a large deep skillet like mine, a wide pot will do the trick. Make sure your skillet or pot has a lid and is big enough to hold the potatoes.

2. SLOW COOKER TURKEY CHILI

On a cold winter evening, nothing warms you up like a big bowl of chili. Although delicious by itself, you can top it with a little organic nonfat Greek yogurt or some fresh avocado. High salt foods may aggravate your symptoms by promoting fluid retention. In this recipe, you can reduce the sodium content by using fresh jalapenos and choosing low sodium canned beans or using beans cooked from dry.

Yield: SERVES 8-10

Prep time: 10 MINUTES

Cook time: 4-6 HOURS

INGREDIENTS:

- 1 tablespoon olive oil

- 1 lb 99% lean ground turkey

- 1 medium onion, diced

- 1 red pepper, chopped

- 1 yellow pepper, chopped

- 2 (15 oz) cans tomato sauce

- 2 (15 oz) cans petite diced tomatoes

- 2 (15 oz) cans black beans, rinsed and drained

- 2 (15oz) cans red kidney beans, rinsed and drained

- 1 (16 oz) jar deli-sliced tamed jalapeno peppers, drained

- 1 cup frozen corn

- 2 tablespoons chili powder

- 1 tablespoon cumin

- Salt and black pepper, to taste

- Optional toppings: green onions, shredded cheese, avocado, sour cream/ Greek yogurt

DIRECTIONS:

1. Heat the oil in a skillet over medium heat. Place turkey in the skillet, and cook until brown. Pour turkey into slow cooker.

2. Add the onion, peppers, tomato sauce, diced tomatoes, beans, jalapeños, corn, chili powder, and cumin. Stir and season with salt and pepper.

3. Cover and cook on High for 4 hours or low for 6 hours. Serve with toppings, if desired.

3. BAKED TILAPIA WITH PECAN ROSEMARY TOPPING

Tilapia is a good source of selenium, a mineral shown to help improve arthritis symptoms. What's great about this recipe is that it's quick enough for a weeknight dinner with the family, but can also be served as a fancier dish. If avoiding gluten, choose gluten-free breadcrumbs for this recipe. If you are not a tilapia eater, trout or cod would work well in this recipe.

Prep time: 15 mins

Cook time: 18 mins

Total time: 35 mins

Serves: 4

INGREDIENTS

- ? cup chopped raw pecans
- ? cup panko breadcrumbs
- 2 tsp chopped fresh rosemary
- ½ tsp (packed) brown sugar
- ? tsp salt
- 1 pinch cayenne pepper
- 1½ tsp olive oil
- 1 egg white
- 4 (4 oz. each) tilapia fillets

INSTRUCTIONS

1. Preheat oven to 350 degrees F.

2. In a small baking dish, stir together pecans, breadcrumbs, brown sugar, salt and cayenne pepper. Add the olive oil and toss to coat the pecan mixture.

3. Bake until the pecan mixture is light golden brown, 7 to 8 minutes.

4. Increase the heat to 400 degrees F. Coat a large glass baking dish with

cooking spray.

5. In a shallow dish, whisk the egg white. Working with one tilapia at a time, dip the fish in the egg white and then the pecan mixture, lightly coating each side. Place the fillets in the prepared baking dish.

6. Press the remaining pecan mixture into the top of the tilapia fillets.

7. Bake until the tilapia is just cooked through, about 10 minutes. Serve.

4. ITALIAN-STYLE STUFFED RED PEPPERS

Instead of a tomato-based pasta sauce, this recipe uses red peppers, which are full of vitamin C and beta carotene.

INGREDIENTS

- 1 lb Lean ground turkey (Or lean ground beef)

- 3 Red bell peppers

- 2 cups Spaghetti sauce

- 1 tsp Basil/oregano seasoning (or any blend of italian herbs)

- 1tsp Garlic powder (or 1 garlic clove, pressed)

- 1/2 tsp Salt and pepper

- 1/2 cup Frozen chopped spinach (or veggie of choice) or (de-thawed and squeezed dry with paper towel)

- 2 tbs Grated parmesan cheese + 6 tbs to garnish over the top of each pepper

- Optional 1 tsp (or 1 packet) low calorie sweetener of choice to put in the sauce (I like my sauce slightly sweet)

METHOD

The estimated total time to make this recipe is 35-40 Minutes.

1. Pre-heat oven to 450 degrees. Line baking sheet with foil, (for easy clean up), coat with non-stick cooking spray. Wash red peppers, and cut around the stem to remove.

2. Remove the stems.

3. Cut peppers in half length-wise, and remove the seeds and ribs inside the peppers. Set peppers on baking pan.

4. Meanwhile, cook ground turkey in a large non-stick pan over medium-high heat. Stir and break up the turkey while it's cooking. When turkey is almost completely cooked through, add the sauce and seasonings to the pan. Stir and continue to cook until the turkey is completely cooked (when it is no longer pink). Add the spinach and parmesan and stir until everything is well combined.

5. Scoop 1/2 cup of the turkey mixture into each pepper.

6. Sprinkle 1 tbs parmesan over each pepper (or another low fat shredded cheese, such as mozzarella).

7. Bake for 20-30 minutes, or until cheese is melted, and lightly golden brown.

8. Remove from the oven, let cool, and enjoy!!!

5. DINNER: LEMON HERB SALMON AND ZUCCHINI

Steaming fish and poultry is a great way to lock in flavor, moisture, vitamins, and minerals. Be sure to serve the fish with some of the steaming liquid, as the liquid will soak up the flavor from the salmon and vegetables.

INGREDIENTS:

- 4 zucchini, chopped

- 2 tablespoons olive oil

- Kosher salt and freshly ground black pepper, to taste

For The Salmon

- 2 tablespoons brown sugar, packed

- 2 tablespoons freshly squeezed lemon juice

- 1 tablespoon Dijon mustard

- 2 cloves garlic, minced

- 1/2 teaspoon dried dill

- 1/2 teaspoon dried oregano

- 1/4 teaspoon dried thyme

- 1/4 teaspoon dried rosemary

- Kosher salt and freshly ground black pepper, to taste

- 4 (5-ounce) salmon fillets

- 2 tablespoons chopped fresh parsley leaves

DIRECTIONS:

1. Preheat oven to 400 degrees F. Lightly oil a baking sheet or coat with nonstick spray.

2. In a small bowl, whisk together brown sugar, lemon juice, Dijon, garlic, dill, oregano, thyme and rosemary; season with salt and pepper, to taste. Set aside.

3. Place zucchini in a single layer onto the prepared baking sheet. Drizzle with olive oil and season with salt and pepper, to taste. Add salmon in a single layer and brush each salmon filet with herb mixture.

4. Place into oven and cook until the fish flakes easily with a fork, about 16-18 minutes.*

5. Serve immediately, garnished with parsley, if desired.

6. DINNER: SWEET POTATO BLACK BEAN BURGERS

These burgers are so fantastic, you may just want to give up eating beef patties. Load up on vitamin C and beta carotene from the sweet potatoes and easily digestible nutrients from the sprouts.

Slightly spicy veggie burgers made with black beans, sweet potatoes, and quinoa. Topped with a delicious sour cream avocado-cilantro crema!

INGREDIENTS

- 1/2 cup quinoa

- 1 can black beans, rinsed and drained

- 1 large sweet potato

- 1/2 cup diced red onion

- 2 cloves garlic, minced

- 1/2 cup chopped cilantro

- 1/2 jalapeno, seeded and diced

- 1 teaspoon cumin

- 2 teaspoons spicy cajun seasoning

- 1/4 gluten free oat flour (regular oat flour or oat bran will work)

- salt and pepper, to taste

- olive oil or coconut oil, for cooking

- 6 whole grain hamburger buns (gluten free, if desired)

- Sprouts

For Avocado-Cilantro Crema:

- 1/2 large ripe avocado, diced

- 1/4 cup low-fat sour cream or plain greek yogurt

- 2 tablespoons chopped cilantro

- 1 teaspoon lime juice

- dash of hot sauce, if desired

- salt, to taste

INSTRUCTIONS

1. To cook quinoa: Rinse quinoa with cold water in mesh strainer. In a medium saucepan, bring 1 cup of water to a boil. Add in quinoa and bring mixture to a boil. Cover, reduce heat to low and let simmer for 15 minutes or until quinoa has absorbed all of the water. Remove from heat and fluff quinoa with fork; place in large bowl and set aside to cool for about 10 minutes. You should have about 1 1/2 cups of quinoa.

2. Poke sweet potato several times with a fork and place in microwave for about 3-4 minutes or until it is soft and cooked thoroughly. Do not overcook or the sweet potato will harden. Alternatively you can roast the sweet potatoes in the oven at 400 degrees F for 30 minutes or until fork tender. Remove skin when done cooking and cooled.

3. In bowl of food processor, add beans, cooked sweet potato, red onion, cilantro, garlic, cumin, cajun seasoning, and pulse until almost smooth, scraping down the sides of the processor when necessary. Transfer mixture to bowl and combine with quinoa. Add salt and pepper to taste - and possibly more cajun seasoning if you'd like. Mix in oat bran/oat flour, but only enough so that you are able to shape patties. (You shouldn't need more than 1/3 cup).

4. Divide into 6 patties (about 1/2 cup each) and place on parchment paper on baking sheet; refrigerate for at least 30 minutes to help patties bind together.

5. To make avocado-cilantro crema: In bowl of food processor, place sour cream, diced avocado, cilantro, and lime juice.

6. Process until smooth. Add salt to taste. Place in fridge until ready to serve burgers.

7. To cook burgers: Heat skillet over medium-high heat. Spray pan with coconut/olive/canola oil cooking spray. Place in skillet and pan-fry about 3-4 minutes on each side, or until golden brown. Serve with buns, sprouts, crema and desired toppings.

7. TURKEY AND QUINOA BELL PEPPERS

Stuffed peppers are a 1950s classic, but this recipe gives it a modern overhaul. Instead of packing the stuffing with calorie- busting bread, use quinoa, one of the world's most powerful superfoods. Skip the green peppers and go for red, yellow, or orange peppers for a sweeter taste.

INGREDIENTS:

- 3 large yellow peppers

- 1.25lb extra lean ground turkey

- 1 C diced mushrooms

- 1/4 C diced sweet onion

- 1 C chopped fresh spinach

- 2 teaspoons minced garlic

- 1 C (1 8oz can) tomato sauce

- 1 C chicken broth

- 1 C dry quinoa

- Optional – cheese of choice. I used pepper jack on half and an Italian cheese blend on the ones for the kids.

DIRECTIONS:

1. In a small saucepan, start the quinoa and cook according to package directions (usually about 15 minutes).

2. While the quinoa cooks, saute the vegetables in a pan with a little butter or olive oil.

3. Then after about 5 minutes or so, add the ground turkey and garlic to the vegetables. Cook over medium heat. Once the turkey is mostly cooked though, add in the tomato sauce and about half of the chicken broth. Let

simmer until the turkey is fully cooked and some of the excess liquid has cooked off.

4. Preheat the oven to 400.

5. While the turkey mixture simmers, prep your bell peppers. Wash the peppers, cut them in half, and remove the stem & seeds. Spray a 9×13 baking pan with cooking spray and place the cut bell peppers in the pan (open side up).

6. Once the quinoa is done cooking, dump it into the pan with the turkey & vegetables. Stir together. Then, stuff each bell pepper with the mixture. Make sure they are nice & full! If you're opting for cheese, then top with just enough cheese to barely cover the mixture (if you put too much on, it will get super messy in the oven!). Pour the rest of the chicken broth into the base of the pan (so around the peppers, not over them).

7. Cover with foil and bake at 400 for about 30-35 minutes. Serve warm & eat up!

8. SWEET POTATOES WITH CINNAMON CHICKEN AND CASHEWS

Give these sweet potatoes a flavorful kick by adding some cinnamon-seasoned chicken and cashews. Dried cherries and raisins also elevate the texture in this topped potato to a perfect savory-sweet terriroty.

INGREDIENTS

- 6 Perfect Roasted Sweet Potatoes

- 1 tablespoon olive oil

- 1/4 cup finely chopped celery

- 1/4 cup dried tart cherries

- 1/4 cup golden raisins

- 3 tablespoons orange juice

- 1/4 teaspoon ground cinnamon

- 1/8 teaspoon ground red pepper

- 1/8 teaspoon kosher salt

- 2 cups shredded skinless, boneless rotisserie chicken breast

- 1/2 cup dry-roasted cashews, unsalted

- 1/4 cup thinly

- sliced green onions

HOW TO MAKE IT

Step 1

Preheat oven to 400°. Bake potatoes according to recipe instructions.

Step 2

Heat a large nonstick skillet over medium heat. Add oil; swirl to coat. Add celery; cook 2 minutes, stirring frequently. Add cherries and next 5 ingredients (through salt); cook 1 minute. Stir in chicken and cashews; cook 2 minutes. Sprinkle with onions. Top potatoes with chicken mixture.

9. FEEL-GOOD PINEAPPLE SMOOTHIE

Yield: 1 Serving

This Feel-Good Pineapple Smoothie recipe is made of a delicious mix of ingredients that also have anti-inflammatory benefits.

Total Time: 5 Mins

Prep Time: 5 Mins

Cook Time: 0 Mins

INGREDIENTS:

- 1 ½ cups frozen pineapple chunks

- 1 orange, peeled

- 1 cup coconut water

- 1 tablespoon finely-chopped fresh ginger (or 1/4 teaspoon ground ginger)

- 1 teaspoon chia seeds, plus extra for garnishing

- 1 teaspoon McCormick Ground Turmeric

- 1/4 teaspoon ground black pepper

DIRECTIONS:

1. Add all ingredients to a blender. Pulse until smooth.

2. Serve immediately, garnished with extra chia seeds if desired.

Difficulty: Easy

10. SHEET PAN HONEY BALSAMIC SALMON WITH BRUSSELS SPROUTS

Prep time: 5 mins

Cook time: 25 mins

Total time: 30 mins

INGREDIENTS

- 4 4-6oz salmon filets (skin on)

- 16 oz. brussels sprouts, halved

- 1 bunch on asparagus, trimmed and cut in half

- 16 oz. bag of baby potatoes

- ½ red onion, cubes

- 1 cup cherry tomatoes

- 2 tablespoons olive oil

- 2 tablespoons honey

- 3 tablespoons balsamic vinegar

- 1 tablespoon dijon mustard

- 1 garlic clove, minced

- 1 teaspoon fresh thym

INSTRUCTIONS

1. Preheat oven to 450.

2. In a small bowl, add honey, balsamic vinegar, dijon mustard, garlic, fresh thyme, and salt. Using a whisk, mix together to combine. Set aside.

3. To a large bowl, add brussels sprouts, asparagus, baby potatoes, red onion, cherry tomatoes and olive oil. Add 3 tablespoons of the honey balsamic mixture.

4. Using your hands, toss all of the vegetables to coat them with the sauce.

5. Spread vegetables out on baking sheet in a single layer.

6. Bake for 10 minutes.

7. Remove from oven.

8. Place salmon filets, skin side down, on top of the vegetables 1" apart.

9. Brush the salmon with the honey balsamic mixture.

10. Place baking sheet back in the oven and bake another 10 minutes.

11. After that switch to broiler HIGH for 3-4 minutes to brown up the top of the salmon.

12. Remove from oven and serve

Nutrition Information

Serving size: 1 salmon filet + veggies Calories: 488 Fat: 12 g Saturated fat: 2 g Carbohydrates: 57 g Sugar: 15 g Sodium: 697 mg Fiber: 6 g Protein: 36 g Cholesterol: 75 mg

11. SHRIMP BOK CHOY AND TURMERIC SOUP

Prep time: 20 mins

Cook time: 30 mins

Total time: 50 mins

Packed full of delicious and healthy ingredients like turmeric, bok choy and shrimp for a healthy gluten free soup recipe. his recipe is gluten, dairy, nut, egg, and soy free, suits the autoimmune protocol (AIP) and paleo diets.

Recipe type: Soup

Serves: 4

INGREDIENTS

- 1 tablespoon Extra Virgin Olive Oil

- 1 large Onion, chopped

- 6 Garlic Cloves, minced

- 1½ teaspoon Salt, plus additional for serving

- 1 teaspoon Ground Black Pepper, plus additional for serving (optional for AIP)

- 1 teaspoon Turmeric

- 6 cups Chicken Broth

- 2 Carrots, sliced

- 1 pound Shitake Mushrooms, stems removed and sliced into ½ inch pieces

- 6 heads Baby Bok Choy, bottoms chopped off

- 1 pound Shrimp

INSTRUCTIONS

1. Heat the oil in a stock pot or dutch oven over medium heat.

2. Add onions and garlic then sauté for 5 minutes or until translucent.

3. Add in salt, pepper, turmeric, chicken broth, carrots and mushrooms then bring to a boil

4. Reduce heat and then let simmer, covered for 20 minutes.

5. Add bok choy and shrimp in the last 5 minutes of cooking.

6. Add salt and pepper to taste then serve.

You can use frozen shrimp for this recipe but keep in mind that they will dilute the soup a little bit. You may need to add in a littler more salt or pepper. Add it to taste but take care to taste as you go.

12. TURMERIC CHICKPEA CAKES

Serves: 4

Prep & Cook time: 15 minutes

INGREDIENTS:

- 1 small onion

- 2 cloves of garlic

- 1 can rinsed and drained chickpeas (or 1 1/2 cups pre-cooked)

- small bunch of fresh parsley, roughly chopped (about 1/4 cup)

- 2 tablespoons potato starch

- 1-2 teaspoons of sea salt

- freshly ground black pepper

- 1 teaspoon turmeric powder

- 1/2 – 1 teaspoon cayenne pepper (optional)

- 2 tablespoons chickpea flour + extra 3 tablespoons for coating

- grape seed oil for cooking

- Garlicky Avocado Cream to serve (recipe will be shared separately soon) (for now you can try this recipe for Avocado Lime

- Cream and omit the lime and add 1/2 minced garlic clove instead)

DIRECTIONS:

1. In a large cast iron pan, drizzle in a little grape seed oil and fry the onion and garlic until slightly golden but not burned. Remove from heat and allow to cool.

2. In a food processor, process the chickpeas until they turn to a slightly textured paste, be sure to turn off the food processor and scrape down

the sides to get all the chickpeas ground up. Add in onion and garlic, salt, pepper, turmeric and cayenne pepper and mix to fully combine. Turn the food processor off and stir in the chopped parsley.

(If you do have kids, I would omit the cayenne pepper entirely as most kids are not into spicy foods. Or divide the batch into two and season them differently for kiddos and adults.)

3. Take a large plate and sprinkle a few tablespoons of chickpea flour onto it. Using a spoon, scoop some of the mixture with onto your hands and shape into a ball, the size of a golf ball, and then press gently to make a patty. Drop into the chickpea flour to coat evenly. If too much flour sticks to the patty then gently dust it off with your fingers or a pastry brush. You should have a very light coating all over the patties/ burgers.

4. Reheat that same large cast iron pan to medium heat. Drizzle in a little more oil and place the patties in to cook. Cook for about 2-3 minutes on each side until the bottom is nicely browned.

5. Serve with a big salad for a healthy lunch or dinner. Or with cut up veggies on the side for kids. Makes a great party small- plates or potluck party dish! Enjoy!

13. SWEET POTATO OVEN FRIES WITH AVOCADO DIP

- **Total:**45 min

- **Prep**: 15 min

- **Cook**: 30 min

- **Yield**: 6 servings

INGREDIENTS

Sweet Potato Fries:

- 2 large sweet potatoes, peeled or unpeeled, cut into 4-inch long and 1/4 to 1/2-inch thick fries

- 2 tablespoons olive oil, or more as needed

- 1 teaspoon paprika

- 1/2 teaspoon chili powder

- 1/2 teaspoon ground coriander

- Coarse ground rock salt and freshly ground black pepper, to taste

- Avocado Dip, recipe follows

Avocado Dip:

- 1 avocado, see Cook's Note*

- 1/3 cup mayonnaise

- 1/3 cup cream cheese

- 1 jalapeno, seeded and chopped.

- 2 scallions, white and light green part only, chopped

- 1 lime, juiced

- Salt and freshly ground black pepper

DIRECTIONS

Sweet Potato Fries:

1. Preheat your oven to 450 degrees F. Line a baking sheet with aluminum foil and set aside.

2. Place the sweet potatoes in a large bowl and toss with olive oil until the sweet potatoes are coated. Add the paprika, chili powder, coriander, salt, and pepper; toss to distribute evenly.

3. Arrange the coated fries in a single layer on the prepared pan. Bake for 20 minutes on the lower rack until the sweet potatoes soften.

4. Transfer the pan to the upper rack of the oven and bake 10 minutes longer, until fries are crispy. Serve with Avocado Dip.

Avocado Dip:

1. Place the avocado, mayonnaise, cream cheese, jalapeno, scallions, and lime juice into a blender or small food processor.

2. Blend for 1 minute or until you have a smooth paste. Season with salt and pepper, to taste. Serve as a dip for the Sweet Potato Oven Fries.

14. ANTI-INFLAMMATORY CACAO GRANOLA RECIPE

INGREDIENTS

- 3 cups rolled oats

- 1 cup unsweetened shredded coconut

- 1 cup raw walnuts (or any other nuts you have on hand)

- ½ cup chia, flax, or hemp seeds (I like a combination)

- ½ teaspoon sea salt

- ½ cup unsweetened cacao or cocoa powder

- 2/3 cup melted coconut oil

- ½ teaspoon vanilla extract

- 1/2 cup honey (agave or maple syrup if vegan)

- 1/3 cup coconut sugar (or light brown sugar)

- 1/4 cup chopped chocolate (optional for extra decadence)

INSTRUCTIONS

1. Preheat oven to 325 degrees Fahrenheit.

2. In a large bowl, stir together the oats, coconut, walnuts, seeds, salt, and cacao. In a medium bowl, whisk together the coconut oil, vanilla, honey, and coconut sugar until smooth. Pour coconut oil mixture over the oat mixture and stir until oats are coated. I find using two rubber spatulas at the same time to mix the ingredients works best. If you like your granola very clumpy, add more honey.

3. Coat one large or two small rimmed baking sheet(s) with cooking spray or rub with a little more coconut oil. Press granola into the bottom of the prepared baking sheet and bake for 15 minutes. Stir and bake another 10-15 minutes. Cool completely in the pan without stirring. Granola will

crisp up, clump, and harden as it cools. Gently stir in chocolate chunks, if desired.

4. Store in an airtight container.

4. Serve over milk and topped with raspberries or bananas. Yum!

Yield: Makes about 6 cups

Prep Time: 10 mins.

Servings: 8

15. CRISPY TURMERIC ROASTED CHICKPEAS RECIPE

Replace the croutons on your salad with a tastier, more nutritious option, or enjoy these turmeric roasted chickpeas alone as a snack.

INGREDIENTS

- 2 15-ounce cans organic chickpeas

- ½ teaspoon coriander

- 2 tablespoons organic turmeric

- 1 teaspoon garam masala

- ½ teaspoon salt

- ½ teaspoon pepper

- ½ teaspoon fenugreek

- 2 tablespoons avocado oil

DIRECTIONS

1. Preheat oven to 400 degrees.

2. Drain chickpeas in a colander, and rinse with water. Spread out chickpeas on a piece of paper towel, and use another one to pat dry. Let air dry for about five minutes. While the chickpeas are drying, mix the dry ingredients in a separate bowl.

3. Transfer the chickpeas to a cookie sheet, and coat with avocado oil. Mix, and put in the oven. After twenty minutes, coat chickpeas with the spice mix and put back in the oven for ten to fifteen more minutes.

4. Remove from oven and let cool before serving. Store in an airtight container.

EAT YOUR ANTI-INFLAMMATORY FRUITS AND VEGGIES!

Fruits and vegetables are vital components to the anti-inflammatory lifestyle. Eating copious amounts of the right types of these disease-fighting foods will allow you to improve your health, feel better, look better, and have more energy! Countless studies have shown eating fruits and vegetables decreases your risk of heart disease, various cancers, diabetes, and numerous other chronic diseases. Your first step is to begin adding non-starchy vegetables to your meals in large quantities. Since 4 cups of green leafy vegetables such as spinach only contain around 30 calories, gaining unhealthy weight from these sources is not an issue! The only vegetables to be generally avoided are starchy tubers, such as potatoes, sweet potatoes, and yams, as these are high glycemic foods that can cause large spikes in blood sugar. However, if you are an athlete training for an event or simply engaging in regular heavy exercise, then these foods can be added to enhance your performance.

Certain types of fruits are better sources of energy than others. Glycemic index and glycemic load are two concepts that have been popularized in the last several years, and are very important to understanding what foods you should be eating. The glycemic index measures how fast a particular food triggers a rise in blood sugar. The higher the amount of glucose or fructose in a food, the fast it breaks down and causes a rise in blood sugar and insulin levels. Grains and starches are simply long chains of glucose held together by carbon bonds. As a result, they break down very quickly and rapidly enter the blood, causing spikes in blood sugar and insulin. Fruits and vegetables, on the other hand, are between 30 and 70 percent fructose, another type of sugar. Fructose converts very slowly to glucose in the liver, so it causes a much smaller insulin response. The insoluble fiber found in fruits and vegetables also acts to further slow down the entrance of fructose into the bloodstream. The total glycemic load of a meal is also important. If a high glycemic food, such as a banana is consumed with a low glycemic food such as a chicken breast, the effect on insulin levels will be much less drastic than if the banana was eaten alone.

Now you can see why eating a potato or piece of bread, which are 100 percent glucose, causes a greater insulin spike than pure table sugar, which is half glucose and half fructose. This is why the concept of glycemic load is even more important, because it takes into account not only the rate at which a food enters the bloodstream, but the amount of calories it contains.

This is very important because some foods have a very high total glycemic index, but do not contain many calories, so their glycemic load is relatively low. For example, a bagel and a serving of watermelon both have a glycemic index of 72, while the glycemic load of the fruit is a mere 4 compared to 25 for the bagel! The higher the glycemic load of your diet, the more insulin your body is producing. A study at Harvard Medical School actually found the higher glycemic load of your diet; the more likely you are to develop obesity, heart disease and diabetes. Clearly, this is an incredibly important concept that must be considered when deciding what foods to eat.

The great thing about the anti-inflammatory method of eating we teach our patients is naturally low glycemic. It should come as no surprise that eating the foods we were designed to eat results in a healthy insulin response, not the jarring ups and downs in mood, energy and overall health that eating a pro-inflammatory diet can cause. For example, a person who is overweight with Type II diabetes will have very different needs, even in regards to the type of fruits and vegetables they are eating, than a competitive tri-athlete burning thousands of calories a day. It cannot be emphasized enough that this program is specific to your needs, not a one-size-fits-all approach. In the Resources section of your manual we have included tables with the glycemic index and load of many common foods as well as recipes using low glycemic foods.

CONCLUSION

Inflammation itself is not a bad thing – it is a normal part of the body's healing system, needed to repair injuries or defend against infection. The problem is when we get generalized or uncontrolled inflammation in the body. Many people believe that the recipes may be a major factor in this.

The inflammatory process in our body is regulated by hormones, which can either increase or reduce the level of inflammation. However, the foods that we eat can dramatically affect these hormone levels, and thus activate or inhibit inflammation in the body.

Anti Inflammatory recipes are vital in alleviating inflammtions in the body. If you are suffering from an inflammatory disease, it would also be wise to avoid pro-inflammatory foods that might increase your pain and inflammation.

Foods to avoid include any junk food and fast food, especially trans-fats and saturated fats. Too much saturated fat means too much arachidonic acid which although essential in the right amounts can be responsible for making your inflammation worse if you consume too much.

Diets high in sugar have also been associated with inflammation and so should be avoided. Another possible cause for concern is foods that come from the deadly nightshade family. Foods such as potatoes, tomatoes and eggplant have been known to aggravate the pain of inflammation.

Adjusting your diet in this way is the first line of defence for any anti-inflammatory regime. Such dietary changes ideally, need to be initiated early on in the disease if they are to have any noticeable effect.

Fortunately there is a growing understanding of how different foods can affect inflammation in the body. This diet is designed to reduce inflammation in the body and promote good health.

The first principle of the anti-inflammatory recipe is that we need a balance of foods. That means eating plenty of fruits and vegetables and as little processed food as possible, and that each meal should contain a mix of carbohydrates, protein and fat.

www.ingramcontent.com/pod-product-compliance
Lightning Source LLC
Chambersburg PA
CBHW050837260726
48660CB00006B/2298